Do you know your Husband

ONE QUESTION A DAY FOR YOU & ME

I0465924

Answer all the following questions honestly! At the end of each category is a score sheet. Read the questions and your answers to your partner and find out how well you did!
Good luck!

Childhood

Answer all the following questions honestly! And at the end of each category is a score sheet, read the questions and your answers to your partner and find out how well you did! Good luck!

♥ What was his first pet?

_____ .

♥ Did your partner have a funny nickname when he was a child? What was it?

YES ☐   NO ☐ _____ .

♥ How did your partner spend his summer as a child?

_____ .

♥ Something that he's always wanted when he was a child but never had.

_____ .

♥ What's his astrological sign?

_____ .

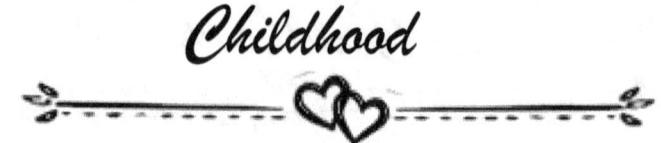

Childhood

Answer all the following questions honestly! And at the end of each category is a score sheet, read the questions and your answers to your partner and find out how well you did! Good luck!

♥ What was his birth order? (Ex. first-born, second-born, etc.)

_____ .

♥ What are his pet peeves?

_____ .

♥ What did his parents taught him that he appreciates now?

_____ .

♥ What is his fondest memory as a child?

_____ .

♥ When your partner was a child, what did he want to be when he grows up?

_____ .

Childhood

Answer all the following questions honestly! And at the end of each category is a score sheet, read the questions and your answers to your partner and find out how well you did! Good luck!

💜 What is his most favorite thing about his childhood?

_____ .

💜 What was the breed and name of his childhood pet?

_____ .

💜 What was the name of his elementary school?

_____ .

💜 What was the ambition of your partner when he was young?

_____ .

💜 Did he ever go to summer camp?

YES ☐   NO ☐

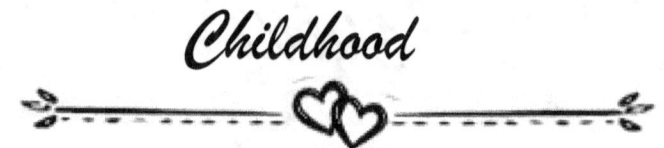

Childhood

Answer all the following questions honestly! And at the end of each category is a score sheet, read the questions and your answers to your partner and find out how well you did! Good luck!

♥ Would he rather spend a day with your parents or his parents?

_____ .

♥ Are his parents still together?

YES ☐ **NO** ☐

♥ Did he play any sports when he was growing up? What kind of sports?

YES ☐ **NO** ☐ _____

_____

_____

♥ What was his least favorite subject in school?

_____ .

♥ Has he ever performed on stage? What did he do?

YES ☐ **NO** ☐ _____ .

Childhood

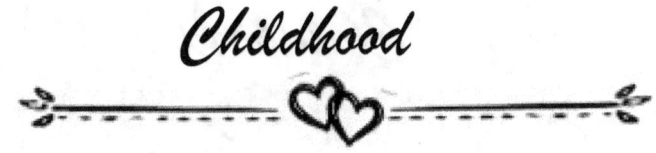

Answer all the following questions honestly! And at the end of each category is a score sheet, read the questions and your answers to your partner and find out how well you did! Good luck!

♥ Has he ever been a part of student government?

YES ☐   NO ☐

♥ Did he get an allowance as a child?

_____.

♥ What are some chores that he had to do when he was growing up?

_____   _____

_____   _____

♥ Did he ever have a favorite restaurant when he was a child? If so, name it.

YES ☐   NO ☐ _____.

♥ Who was his oldest friend?

_____.

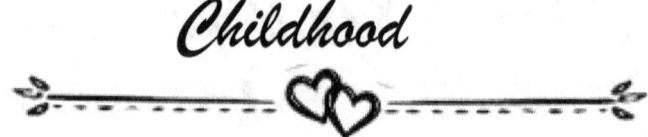

Childhood

Answer all the following questions honestly! And at the end of each category is a score sheet, read the questions and your answers to your partner and find out how well you did! Good luck!

♥ What is the worst trouble that he got into as a child?

_____.

♥ What is one club that he participated in at school?

_____.

♥ What was his favorite subject in school?

_____.

♥ Does he have any nieces or nephews? Name 3 of them.

YES ☐ NO ☐ _____

_____

_____

♥ What town did he grow up in?

_____.

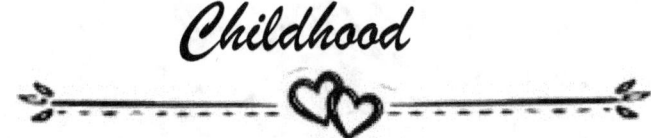

Childhood

Answer all the following questions honestly! And at the end of each category is a score sheet, read the questions and your answers to your partner and find out how well you did! Good luck!

❤ What is his least favorite thing about his childhood?

_____ .

❤ What year did he graduate from high school?

_____ .

❤ Was he brought up in a certain religion?

YES ☐   NO ☐

❤ Has he ever had to repeat a grade in school?

YES ☐   NO ☐

❤ Does your partner consider himself more like his mother or his father in terms of personality? In what way?

_____ .

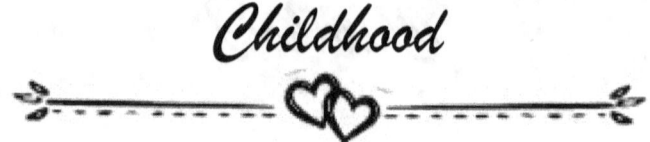

Childhood

Reminder: Any question you answered incorrectly is an opportunity to learn more things about your partner. The questions were designed for couples who have been together for several years.

QUIZ RESULTS

YOUR SCORE

Favorites

Answer all the following questions honestly! And at the end of each category is a score sheet, read the questions and your answers to your partner and find out how well you did! Good luck!

♥ Is your partner very close to your family?

YES ☐   NO ☐

♥ At what age did your partner last live with his parents?

_____ .

♥ Can you list the relatives your partner cannot stand?

_____   _____

_____   _____

♥ Can you name two or more of your partner's grandparents?

_____   _____

_____   _____

♥ Did he go to private or public school?

_____

_____ .

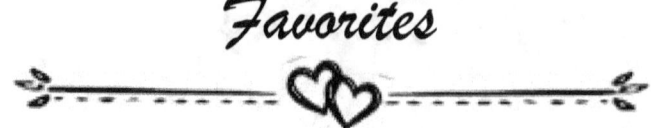

Favorites

Answer all the following questions honestly! And at the end of each category is a score sheet, read the questions and your answers to your partner and find out how well you did! Good luck!

♥ What are the names of your partner's parents?

_____ _____

♥ What are his thoughts on adoption?

_____ .

♥ How's your partner's relationship with his parents?

_____ .

♥ How's your partner's relationship with your family?

_____ .

♥ What is his middle name?

_____ .

Favorites

Answer all the following questions honestly! And at the end of each category is a score sheet, read the questions and your answers to your partner and find out how well you did! Good luck!

♥ What is his mom's maiden name?

_____ .

♥ What are the names of your partner's siblings?

_____   _____

_____   _____

♥ What does his family think of you?

_____ .

♥ What are his parents' jobs?

_____ .

♥ Where do his parents live?

_____ .

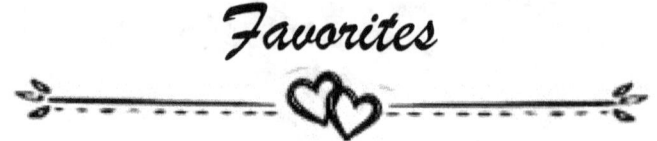

Favorites

Answer all the following questions honestly! And at the end of each category is a score sheet, read the questions and your answers to your partner and find out how well you did! Good luck!

♥ When was your partner's birthday?

_____ .

♥ What would you do to make it a perfect Sunday for him?

_____ .

♥ Who are his favorite aunts and uncles? Name them.

_____   _____

_____   _____

♥ Would he rather spend an evening out with his parents or your parents?

_____ .

♥ Is he close to his extended family?

YES ☐   NO ☐

Favorites

Answer all the following questions honestly! And at the end of each category is a score sheet, read the questions and your answers to your partner and find out how well you did! Good luck!

♥ What is his favorite part of your marriage?

_____ .

♥ What is his favorite thing about your personality?

_____ .

♥ What is his favorite time spending habit?

_____ .

♥ What is your partner's favorite fast food restaurant?

_____ .

♥ What is his favorite part of your body?

_____ .

Favorites

Answer all the following questions honestly! And at the end of each category is a score sheet, read the questions and your answers to your partner and find out how well you did! Good luck!

♥ What is your partner's favorite color?

_____ .

♥ What is his favorite sex position?

_____ .

♥ What is his favorite shoe brand?

_____ .

♥ What will your partner say is your favorite food?

_____ .

♥ What's his favorite meal?

_____ .

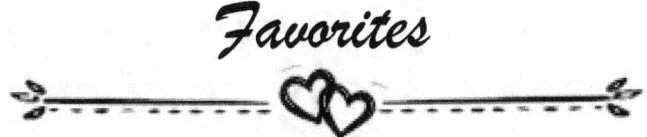

Favorites

Answer all the following questions honestly! And at the end of each category is a score sheet, read the questions and your answers to your partner and find out how well you did! Good luck!

♥ What's his favorite song? And according to him, what is your favorite song?

_____.

♥ What's his favorite time of year?

_____.

♥ What's your partner's favorite flavor of ice cream?

_____.

♥ What's your partner's least favorite body part?

_____.

♥ What is his favorite kind of cake?

_____.

Favorites

Answer all the following questions honestly! And at the end of each category is a score sheet, read the questions and your answers to your partner and find out how well you did! Good luck!

♥ What's your partner's least favorite housework task?

_____ .

♥ What's the name of his favorite celebrity crush?

_____ .

♥ What's your partner's favorite alcoholic drink?

_____ .

♥ What's your partner's favorite clothing brand?

_____ .

♥ What's your partner's favorite music he's listening to these days?

_____ .

16

Favorites

Answer all the following questions honestly! And at the end of each category is a score sheet, read the questions and your answers to your partner and find out how well you did! Good luck!

♥ What's your partner's favorite vacation idea?

_____ .

♥ What's your partner's favorite part of his body?

_____ .

♥ What is your partner's favorite pizza toppings?

_____ .

♥ What's your partner's favorite scent?

_____ .

♥ What's your partner's favorite housework task?

_____ .

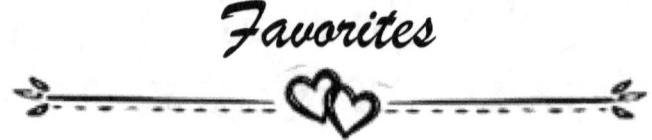

Favorites

Answer all the following questions honestly! And at the end of each category is a score sheet, read the questions and your answers to your partner and find out how well you did! Good luck!

♥ What is your partner's favorite cereal?

_____ .

♥ Who is your partner's favorite fiction character?

_____ .

♥ Who is your partner's favorite music artist?

_____ .

♥ What is his favorite ball game?

_____ .

♥ What is his favorite sandwich?

_____ .

Favorites

Answer all the following questions honestly! And at the end of each category is a score sheet, read the questions and your answers to your partner and find out how well you did! Good luck!

♥ What is his favorite shop?

_____ .

♥ What is his favorite chips flavor?

_____ .

♥ What is his least favorite drink?

_____ .

♥ What is your partner's favorite fruit?

_____ .

♥ What is his favorite board game?

_____ .

Favorites

Reminder: Any question you answered incorrectly is an opportunity to learn more things about your partner. The questions were designed for couples who have been together for several years.

QUIZ RESULTS

YOUR SCORE

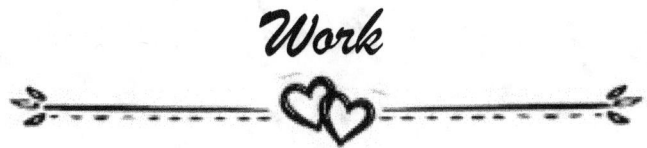

Work

Answer all the following questions honestly! And at the end of each category is a score sheet, read the questions and your answers to your partner and find out how well you did! Good luck!

♥ Does he love his job?

_____ .

♥ Do you know what your partner likes best about her/his work/job?

_____ .

♥ Does he consider art a career?

_____ .

♥ What is the worst job he ever had?

_____ .

♥ What is his dream job?

_____ .

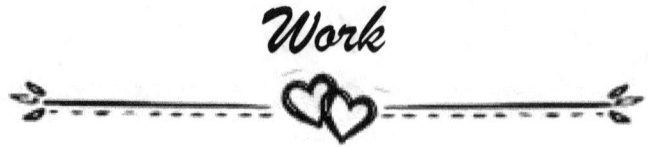

Work

Answer all the following questions honestly! And at the end of each category is a score sheet, read the questions and your answers to your partner and find out how well you did! Good luck!

♥ What does he want out of his career?

_____ .

♥ What makes him feel overwhelmed at work?

_____ .

♥ Who is his biggest role model?

_____ .

♥ Who was his first employer?

_____ .

♥ What was your happiest moment at work?

_____ .

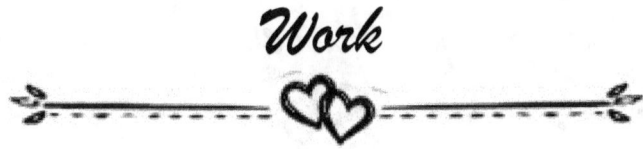

Work

Reminder: Any question you answered incorrectly is an opportunity to learn more things about your partner. The questions were designed for couples who have been together for several years.

QUIZ RESULTS

YOUR SCORE

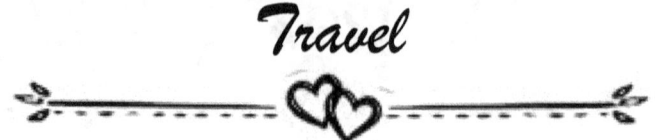

Travel

Answer all the following questions honestly! And at the end of each category is a score sheet, read the questions and your answers to your partner and find out how well you did! Good luck!

♥ Name a country your partner would love to visit.

_____ .

♥ Where did he bring you on your first date?

_____ .

♥ Do you know three places your partner would love to visit?

YES ☐   NO ☐   _____

_____

_____

♥ If he could drive one car for the rest of his life, what would it be?

_____ .

♥ What are some cities or countries that he absolutely would never live in?

_____ .

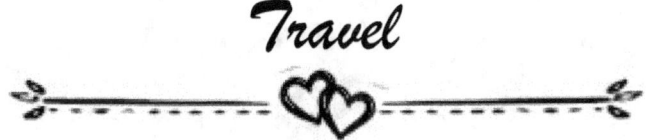

Travel

Answer all the following questions honestly! And at the end of each category is a score sheet, read the questions and your answers to your partner and find out how well you did! Good luck!

♥ What is the oddest location you've ever shared a kiss?

_____ .

♥ What was the best vacation you've ever taken together?

_____ .

♥ What's his idea of a romantic vacation?

_____ .

♥ Where did he last fly to?

_____ .

♥ Where does he dream of going?

_____ .

Travel

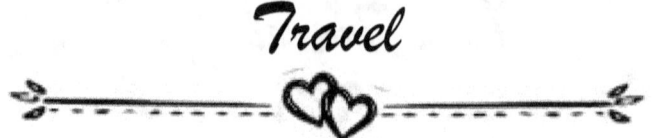

Answer all the following questions honestly! And at the end of each category is a score sheet, read the questions and your answers to your partner and find out how well you did! Good luck!

♥ Where does your husband to be want to go on honeymoon?   (Skip if not applicable)

_____ .

♥ Where in the world he wouldn't like to be right now?

_____ .

♥ Which place would he no longer come back for vacation?

_____ .

♥ Does he do the planning for a vacation?
   YES ☐   **NO** ☐

♥ What's one place that he's always wanted to visit?

_____ .

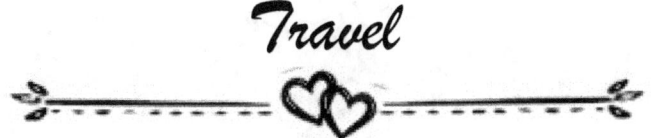

Travel

Answer all the following questions honestly! And at the end of each category is a score sheet, read the questions and your answers to your partner and find out how well you did! Good luck!

♥ Where would he want to travel the most?

_____ .

♥ What are 3 places that he's been to and would love to visit again?

_____ .

♥ Does he prefer to travel alone or with a group?

_____ .

♥ Does he prefer to travel by car, plane, or train?

_____ .

♥ Has he ever been on a cruise?

_____ .

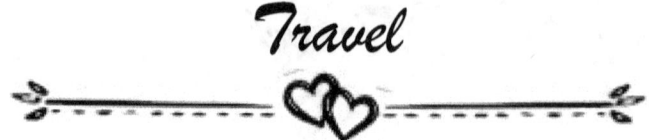

Travel

Answer all the following questions honestly! And at the end of each category is a score sheet, read the questions and your answers to your partner and find out how well you did! Good luck!

♥ If his job forced him to take a vacation for 3 days, what do you think he would do?

_____

_____ .

♥ If he could get on a plane to anywhere in the world, where would he go?

_____ .

♥ What is the longest road trip that he's been on?

_____ .

♥ How many countries has he traveled to?

_____ .

♥ Does he love camping?

_____ .

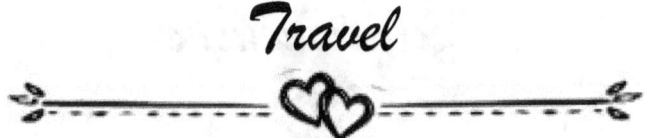

Travel

Reminder: Any question you answered incorrectly is an opportunity to learn more things about your partner. The questions were designed for couples who have been together for several years.

QUIZ RESULTS

YOUR SCORE

Relationships

Answer all the following questions honestly! And at the end of each category is a score sheet, read the questions and your answers to your partner and find out how well you did! Good luck!

♥ Does he have to know all of your friends?

YES ☐   **NO** ☐

♥ How long did it take to plan the wedding? (Skip of not applicable)

_____ .

♥ According to him, what qualities first attracted him to you?

_____ .

♥ How many children does he want?

_____ .

♥ How often would he want to go out on a date with you in a month?

_____ .

Relationships

Answer all the following questions honestly! And at the end of each category is a score sheet, read the questions and your answers to your partner and find out how well you did! Good luck!

♥ The thing he likes the most about you?

_____.

♥ What did he think of you when you first met?

_____.

♥ What is your name on his phonebook?

_____.

♥ What was the last text message he sent you?

_____.

♥ Is he affectionate?

_____.

Relationships

Answer all the following questions honestly! And at the end of each category is a score sheet, read the questions and your answers to your partner and find out how well you did! Good luck!

♥ How old was he when he got her first kiss?

_____ .

♥ Who was his first kiss?

_____ .

♥ Who was his first love?

_____ .

♥ Is he friends with any of his exes?

_____ .

♥ How many exes does he have?

_____ .

Relationships

Answer all the following questions honestly! And at the end of each category is a score sheet, read the questions and your answers to your partner and find out how well you did! Good luck!

♥ What are his thoughts on having children?

_____

_____ .

♥ Can you describe your partner's philosophy of life (how he makes sense of this world)?

_____

_____ .

♥ Does he believe in TRUE love?

YES ☐   NO ☐

♥ Does he think celebrating Valentine's Day is corny?

YES ☐   NO ☐

♥ Does he think confessions make a relationship stronger?

YES ☐   NO ☐

Relationships

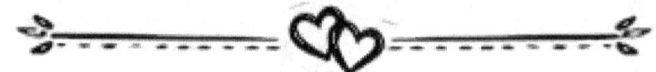

Answer all the following questions honestly! And at the end of each category is a score sheet, read the questions and your answers to your partner and find out how well you did! Good luck!

♥ Does he ever cheated on a lover in a past relationship?

YES ☐   NO ☐

♥ Has an ex-lover invited him to the wedding?

YES ☐   NO ☐

♥ Has he ever pretend he's sleeping just to avoid an argument?

YES ☐   NO ☐

♥ How can he show you that he's listening to you?

_____ .

♥ How did his heart break the first time?

_____ .

Relationships

Answer all the following questions honestly! And at the end of each category is a score sheet, read the questions and your answers to your partner and find out how well you did! Good luck!

♥ How did he propose to you?

_____ .

♥ How often does he want to hear from you?

_____ .

♥ How often would he like to go out on a date night?

_____ .

♥ How did he express his love for you last Valentine's Day?

_____ .

♥ Three things he likes about you.

_____

_____

_____

Relationships

Answer all the following questions honestly! And at the end of each category is a score sheet, read the questions and your answers to your partner and find out how well you did! Good luck!

♥ True/ False? Your significant other was happy with the first gift you ever gave him.

_____.

♥ What are 3 practical ways that he can show his love for you?

_____

_____

_____

♥ Who was his first crush?

_____.

♥ What are his thoughts on Public Display of Affection (PDA)?

_____.

♥ What can he do to keep your love alive?

_____.

Relationships

♥ What comes to his mind when he thinks of your exes?

_____ .

♥ What could he do to make you feel more respected?

_____ .

♥ What drew him to you?

_____ .

♥ What has he learned from watching your friends' relationships progress over the years?

_____ .

♥ What is most important to him in a relationship?

_____ .

Relationships

Answer all the following questions honestly! And at the end of each category is a score sheet, read the questions and your answers to your partner and find out how well you did! Good luck!

♥ Who was his first friend?

_____ .

♥ Who would he say is the boss in the relationship?

_____ .

♥ Is he open with disclosing all his health issues to you all the time?

_____ .

♥ Would he ever say sorry to you even if it's not his fault?

_____ .

♥ Would he relocate for love?

_____ .

Relationships

Answer all the following questions honestly! And at the end of each category is a score sheet, read the questions and your answers to your partner and find out how well you did! Good luck!

♥ Describe his/her ideal date night with you?

_____.

♥ What's his first memory with you?

_____.

♥ What gift that you gave to your partner came as the biggest surprise?

_____.

♥ What is the honeymoon destination that your partner would most likely choose for a second honeymoon?

_____.

♥ What is his biggest pet peeve when it comes to the opposite sex?

_____.

Relationships

Reminder: Any question you answered incorrectly is an opportunity to learn more things about your partner. The questions were designed for couples who have been together for several years.

QUIZ RESULTS

YOUR SCORE

Intimate

Answer all the following questions honestly! And at the end of each category is a score sheet, read the questions and your answers to your partner and find out how well you did! Good luck!

♥ Do you know how many times (in a perfect world) he would like to have sex per week?

_____ .

♥ Is he wild or gentle in bed?

_____ .

♥ Are there sexual things your significant one desires to do to you that you should give him more space to do so? Like licking you, rubbing you, stripping you, sucking you?

_____ .

♥ Can he avoid flirting if someone attractive flirts with him?

_____ .

♥ Does he have sensitive nipples?

_____ .

Intimate

Answer all the following questions honestly! And at the end of each category is a score sheet, read the questions and your answers to your partner and find out how well you did! Good luck!

♥ Do you know precisely how and where your partner likes to be touched? Explain.

YES ☐   NO ☐ _____

_____

_____

♥ Does he call it love making, sex, or the crude f**k word?

_____ .

♥ What time does he love to make love to you?

_____ .

♥ Does he feel you only use him for sex?

_____ .

♥ Did he ever have sex in the great outdoors?

_____ .

42

Intimate

Answer all the following questions honestly! And at the end of each category is a score sheet, read the questions and your answers to your partner and find out how well you did! Good luck!

♥ Do you know three of your partner's sexual fantasies? What are they?

YES ☐ NO ☐ _____

_____

_____

♥ When did he lose his virginity?

_____ .

♥ Does your partner like it when you spank him or grab his butt?

YES ☐ NO ☐

♥ Does he love it when you talk dirty or he likes a neat love making session?

YES ☐ NO ☐

♥ Does he love to flirt with you on the phone?

YES ☐ NO ☐

Intimate

Answer all the following questions honestly! And at the end of each category is a score sheet, read the questions and your answers to your partner and find out how well you did! Good luck!

♥ Does he masturbate?

YES ☐ **NO** ☐

♥ Does he orgasm once in a love making session or multiple times?

YES ☐ **NO** ☐

♥ Does he orgasm too quickly and does he like it that way?

YES ☐ **NO** ☐

♥ Does your partner watch pornography?

YES ☐ **NO** ☐

♥ About how long does it take for your partner to be aroused again for another session of love making?

_____ .

Intimate

Answer all the following questions honestly! And at the end of each category is a score sheet, read the questions and your answers to your partner and find out how well you did! Good luck!

♥ Has your significant one ever complained about you going too fast?

YES ☐   NO ☐

♥ How many sexual partners did he have in the past?

_____ .

♥ Is there anything your partner considers a turn off?

_____ .

♥ Is there anything your partner loves you doing it to him?

_____ .

♥ Did he ever use a sex toy?

YES ☐   NO ☐

Intimate

Answer all the following questions honestly! And at the end of each category is a score sheet, read the questions and your answers to your partner and find out how well you did! Good luck!

♥ Does he have any unaccomplished sexual fantasy? If yes, what is it?

YES ☐   NO ☐ _____.

♥ What does he find sexiest about a person of the opposite sex?

_____.

♥ What does he wear to bed?

_____.

♥ What is that one thing that your partner does to you or on you to show you he wants to make love?

_____.

♥ What is that one thing you do to your partner that arouses him quickly?

_____.

Intimate

Reminder: Any question you answered incorrectly is an opportunity to learn more things about your partner. The questions were designed for couples who have been together for several years.

QUIZ RESULTS

YOUR SCORE

Fun

Answer all the following questions honestly! And at the end of each category is a score sheet, read the questions and your answers to your partner and find out how well you did! Good luck!

♥ Is he a dog or cat lover?

_____ .

♥ Is he good in video games?
YES ☐ **NO** ☐

♥ Has he ever appeared on television? What show?
YES ☐ **NO** ☐ _____ .

♥ Is he a coffee person or a tea person?

_____ .

♥ Does your partner love gadgets?
YES ☐ **NO** ☐

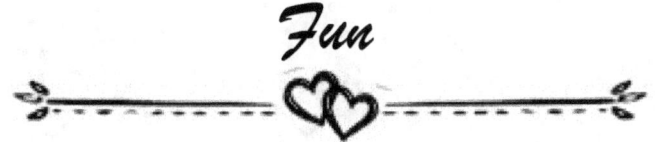

Fun

Answer all the following questions honestly! And at the end of each category is a score sheet, read the questions and your answers to your partner and find out how well you did! Good luck!

♥ Is he a morning person or a night owl?

_____ .

♥ Is he addicted to anything? If yes, to what is he specifically addicted to?

YES ☐   NO ☐ _____ .

♥ Is he an animal lover or would he avoid keeping animals at home?

_____ .

♥ Is there any unique talent that he possesses? What is it?

YES ☐   NO ☐ _____ .

♥ What is the sports team he loves?

_____ .

Fun

Reminder: Any question you answered incorrectly is an opportunity to learn more things about your partner. The questions were designed for couples who have been together for several years.

QUIZ RESULTS

YOUR SCORE

www.ingramcontent.com/pod-product-compliance
Lightning Source LLC
Chambersburg PA
CBHW071241220526
45468CB00002B/958